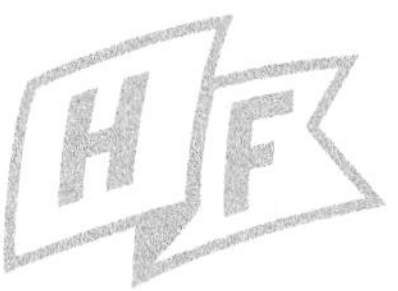

THE JOURNEY TO SELF GIFT

The Four Pillars of a Catholic Fitness Lifestyle

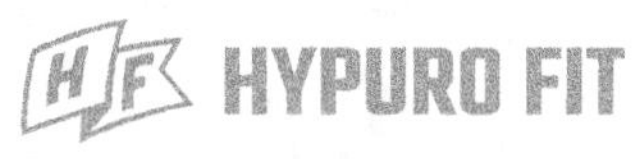

A Hypuro Fit Publication

To the ladies in our lives:
Viva + Carlina
Kathleen, Lucy, + Caeli

It's all for you.

Table of Contents

Hear, O Israel:
The Lord is our God, the Lord alone.
You shall love the Lord your God with
all your heart, and with all your soul,
and with all your might.

- Deut 6:4-5

Introduction:
What's Your "Why"?

*"Those who have a 'why' to live,
can bear with almost any 'how'."*

Viktor Frankl's book *Man's Search for Meaning* has many such gems. As an Austrian psychologist imprisoned for three years in a Nazi concentration camp, he had seen the limits of human endurance and identified having a "why" – a deep underlying motivation based on a sense of direction through finding meaning in one's own life – as one of the indicators of survival within the camps themselves but also as an effective tool for processing the grief afterwards.

We won't be talking about grief and psychotherapy in this book, we'll be talking about Catholic spirituality and fitness. Before that, however, I want to start with a strong emphasis on the importance of a "why". While it's not likely that you or I will experience anything like the Holocaust in our lifetime, a proper "why" is what gives life direction and focus. It's what keeps things from getting off track in turbulent times and, more importantly, what keeps them from getting off track during the good ones. A "why" defines the habits we strive to form, and our habits create a disposition to the good or to the base.

When striving to create consistency in your life there are two components that make up a sturdy habit: motivation and discipline. Motivation sets you on the path to your goal, puts a fire in your belly and fills you with zeal. Discipline keeps you on that track when the going gets tough. We've packed this book with tools for forming a robustly disciplined life but if you're not starting your journey with a proper motivation then your discipline is pointed at nothing and your habits will eventually fall apart.

Generally speaking we don't do things that we aren't motivated to do but in our nexus of motivations there's a hierarchy of importance and dependence. I'm motivated to eat in order to survive but that's dependent on time, meaning I don't eat constantly but at designated intervals (most days at least). However, even the desire to survive defers to greater motivations like defending my wife and children (for whom I'd gladly give my life). I have a motivation to read because of the joy and stimulation that books bring. I have a motivation to spend time with friends because man is a social creature and I'm filled up by the meaningful relationships in my life. The whole myriad of things I'm motivated to do can be grouped under an umbrella of my motivation to find joy. I use this to demonstrate that our small "why's" contribute to more meaningful "why's" and that at the end of it all of it there is one, ultimate "why" that beckons to the whole human race.

This is a book about developing an authentically Catholic fitness lifestyle. It's directed toward Catholics but it is our hope that Christians of all stripes (and all people of good will) can find our message helpful primarily for this reason: the ultimate "why" that drives us forward is perfect union with God.

The difficulty too many of us become mired in is that we're easily distracted by shiny objects. We have a desire to know, love, and serve God but that desire is vague and distant. When momentary excitements flare we follow the trails of entertainment, indulgence, and vanity often to a point of numbness. Then, when we set about our relationship with God through prayer, we experience some distraction or difficulty in starting and abandon the thing altogether! Our motivations are there (to a greater or lesser degree) but our discipline is way off. We're slaves to impulse. Our "why" is not channeled through a proper "how".

The thing I hope you can take away from this book, if nothing else, is to know that we do not advocate for exercise for exercise's sake; we propose the development of an exercise habit as the natural expression of a life oriented toward God and our ultimate "why". We see fitness as an essential part of a fully Catholic lifestyle, something that encapsulates your body, your mind, and your spirit. The way we exercise as Catholics should look different from the secular culture around us. Catholicism is not a set of lifeless ideologies but a living expression of the divine romance that we're all caught up in. It's a relationship that bestows benefits and also makes demands. It's something to be worked at (like any good relationship). A Catholic lifestyle is not just something that happens between your ears, it's a life of declaration; a witness to a *particular* truth! Namely that God loves us more than we could ever hope to be loved and has taken the initiative in bringing us to a home of eternal joy.

Accepting God's invitation means an imitation of his earthly life; it means that, whether we like it or not, a cross is part of the equation. Exercise and bodily discipline are available to us as an arena in which we allow that lesson to be learned in our bodies. It is both education and participation in the purgative component of salvation.

In the following pages we hope to convince you that fitness is an essential part of living out your Christian witness effectively and, when undertaken thoughtfully and intentionally, a sure means of spiritual progression. Like I mentioned at the beginning, it is necessary in this endeavor to marry a deep and meaningful "why" with a consistent and practical "how". Each expression of this relationship will look unique in the same way that mankind is created in a splendid diversity. This is not a road of ease and comfort. It's much better; it's good. If we're honest, we can see that comfort has never been a part of the promise of life.

Know that, as we've penned every page of what you're about to read, we've been lifting you up in prayer. It is our desire that through this you may, in some way, taste the transformation and flourishing that we have experienced in dedicating our time in the gym to God.

In Christ,

Ben + Chase

Pillar One

GIFT OF SELF

Knowing Your Motivation

Something truly remarkable happened in the 70's and 80's, for the first time ever a pope gave a series of lectures on the beauty and glory of the human body. These lectures were given by Pope St. John Paul II and were later referred to collectively as the "Theology of the Body". While this book is definitely NOT a book on the theology of the body, or a commentary on all of the wonderful things that John Paul II said, it is important for us to consider that it is when he started speaking on the theology of the body that we started to see a shift in conversations amongst Catholics in regards to the way we talk about the body.

The body, and sexuality in particular, was no longer a taboo subject that you couldn't touch with a 39 ½ foot pole. Pope John Paul II reclaimed the body for Christ and his Church! He did this by pointing out how good and beautiful the body is and how it's a sign that is supposed to point us back to the love of the Father, Son, and Holy Spirit.

These teachings of JP II were picked up by theologians, priests, and lay people alike. There was energy and enthusiasm because Catholics, especially in America, were being told for the first time that their bodies and sexuality were good, in fact it was *very good*. It was so good, in fact, that it was given to us by God in order to give to others. Our bodies, which make up who we are along with our souls, are meant to be given for service to both God and others. This idea of "self gift" came from an earlier document that JP II references called *Gaudium et Spes* where we read: "man, who is the only creature on earth which God willed for itself, cannot fully find himself except through a *sincere gift* of himself."

Here we find the heart of all of the chaos and anxiety that has been so prevalent in America since the sexual revolution in the 60's and 70's. Everyone desires, with everything that they have, to be loved and to love in return. There is a fire in all of us that longs to burn for the sake of others. Why? Because in some way, we are all seeking self discovery. That's why people who only seek self improvement at the cost of the people around them tend to have broken relationships and lives. If you desire self discovery, but turn it into a narcissistic hunt that ignores everyone else but yourself, then you will never find it. Sure you might find pleasure, but you will never find yourself because that only comes through a "sincere gift of self".

That is hopefully part of the reason why you picked up this book on catholic fitness. We shouldn't fear the body, and, in fact, we should strive to take care of our bodies. On the other hand, as Catholics we also can't give into the temptation of working out and staying active just for the sake of looking good. Looking your best is an awesome perk to staying active and fit, but it can't be the primary factor. It is so easy for vanity and pride to creep in and the enemy is looking for every chance to whisper lies about your body image and comparing yourself to others. We work out in order to prepare ourselves to be a gift to others.

St. Augustine knew this truth first hand. Here is a saint who spent his entire youth focused on one thing: self discovery through the pursuit of knowledge. He learned from all of the local teachers and philosophers until he surpassed them. Thirsty for knowledge and self fulfillment, he traveled to Italy in order to seek the answers to his questions there. He searched and searched and always came up short. He debated and won arguments. For what? Momentary satisfaction. It wasn't until he discovered the Truth found in Jesus Christ and his Church that his heart was finally at rest. As he says in his Confessions: "Thou hast made us for thyself, O Lord, and our heart is restless until it finds its rest in thee"

The discovery that Jesus Christ had desired and pursued him since the day he was born until the day of his conversion triggered something in St. Augustine. He knew that his vain pursuit of knowledge and glory would never satisfy, so he allowed God to use him in order to instruct and evangelize others. He found himself through a sincere gift of self. He later wrote in his Confessions: "What does love look like? It has the hands to help others. It has the feet to hasten to the poor and needy. It has eyes to see misery and want. It has the ears to hear the sighs and sorrows of men. That is what love looks like."

Another famous saint that truly found himself through a sincere gift of self was St. Ignatius of Loyola. Like many young spanish men of his time, St. Ignatius pursued glory and fame by any means. He was so enamored in his pursuit and defense of his own honor that he was even arrested for a nighttime brawl! Like many of us, it took a "cannonball" moment for him to allow God to start influencing his life, literally. While he was leading men into a battle against french soldiers, he was struck in the leg with a cannonball. This effectively ended his career as a soldier and forced him into bed rest for several months.

It was during this time that he asked for books on valor, glory, and chivalry. He was given a book on the saints instead. St. Ignatius had spent his life looking up to feats of heroism on the battlefield, yet in these pages he found himself encountering acts of heroism that were much greater than anything he had ever done in battle. Once he was well enough to leave the hospital St. Ignatius dedicated his life to serving God, his church, and every person he encountered.

Both St. Augustine and St. Ignatius, along with all of the saints, have one crucial mindset in common: self awareness is the first step in the spiritual and moral life. St. Augustine says in his confessions, "This is the very perfection of man, to find out his own imperfections." This might seem contradictory but it is far from it.

If you play any sports, or know someone who has tried learning a new sport, then you know that a key element in improving your game is the ability to identify where you are weakest and work on it. I grew up playing basically every sport. As a young man from Texas it was one of those unspoken rules that every boy at least try all of the usual sports like football, baseball, and basketball. What I learned quickly, however, was that I didn't have much of an arm (I also got hit with a baseball decent amount which didn't impress my 5 year old mind). I wasn't big. I was tall, but not *that* tall. So none of these sports really panned out for me. I eventually discovered a love for tennis. I'm one of those lanky-but-quick guys so this sport worked out nicely.

I spent every free summer day and evening from when I was 10 years old through high school practicing and honing my craft. How did I practice? By working on the things I hadn't mastered yet. For me it was always my backhand. I switched from a two handed grip to a one handed grip in 8th grade, because I thought it looked cooler, and I spent the next 3 years trying to improve it. I even lost tournaments because my opponents would notice it was weak and take advantage. Eventually I figured it out and what was once a weakness turned into one of my favorite shots.

In the moral life there is a similar connection. We all struggle with some kind of sin or vice that our personality or genetic makeup simply tends towards naturally. If we ignore it then it can turn into a deep set vice that does serious harm to ourselves and others. With the help of God's transformative grace though, by striving to overcome our unique shortcomings, we become equipped in a special way to defeat those particular vices and empathize with those who have similar struggles.

For those who have read C.S. Lewis' *The Great Divorce*, the encounter where the lizard of lust is killed and transformed into the stallion of desire illustrates this beautifully. As the man who had been subject to the whisperings of the demon on his shoulder is freed by that creature's death, the very hills of the land sing out *"all natures that were your enemies become slaves to dance before you and backs for you to ride...The strengths that once opposed your will shall be obedient fire in your blood".*

This same logic applies to serving others. St. Ignatius says, rather bluntly, that "The man who sets about making others better is wasting his time, unless he begins with himself." I think we have all had moments where we have corrected someone or became angry at someone who did something wrong only to realize soon afterwards that we also struggle with the very same thing and aren't doing anything to correct it. We can never expect to spread the gospel and to help others grow in virtue if we aren't first working on our own relationship with Jesus every single day.

Everything for St. Augustine and St. Ignatius came down to making sure that they were fully able to give of themselves. The reason we must focus in on our own personal sins and struggles is to get rid of all of the internal and external things that prevent us from being a gift to others. The mistake that some make is that they think that this journey only happens in the mind and soul. But being able to give a "sincere gift of self" requires the whole self, which includes our bodies! Our "true selves" aren't trapped inside of our bodies trying to escape. To be human is to have a soul *and* a body. We aren't angels with only intellects. We are also more than just mere animals with only instincts and simple emotions. The thing that makes us unique as humans is that we are *embodied*. The reason that the resurrection of the body is necessary at the end of time is because we are made to be body and soul. Therefore we must take care of both our body and our soul in order to prepare for eternity.

The world has changed since John Paul II reconquered the body for Christ. There is no longer any excuse for us to fear the body. We know that our bodies are important and that it takes work and effort to reconquer them for the sake of service. That's what this book, and Catholic fitness, is all about, reconquering our bodies for Christ.

Are you ready to learn how?

At the end of every chapter, we'll include short practical tips to help apply the lessons to your daily life. These are suggestions to help get you started and can be augmented to either be more of less difficult depending on where you're at in your journey.

Spiritual Challenge:

For 1 week, wake up 20 minutes before you usually do and pray a Rosary. Offer it up for someone different every day. The first thing you will do every day is make a sacrifice of your sleep and your prayer.

Physical Challenge:

How many push-ups can you do? If you need to put your knees on the ground to do one then cool. If you can do one with your knees off the ground, great. Either way, find the max amount you can do and try to hit that count or beat it every day for a week.

He Conquers Who Conquers Himself

What is the most challenging experience you have ever been through? Maybe it was something mental, like finishing college. The hours you spent working on the 50 page paper, finishing that reading list, or working on that project with a team of people you weren't sure you could trust. Perhaps it was something physical, like making it through basic training in the military or training for a competition. I remember all of the stories my Dad told me of when he was in basic training for the army. He would tell me of all the sleepless nights and going weeks on end without showering (that might sound petty but you try going a month without showering and see how you feel). It might be hard for you to identify one specific time as the most difficult, it is for me, but one of the most challenging, yet grace filled parts of my life was my time as a missionary.

While it would sound cool to say that I went off into the wilderness of the Amazon, or to the parts of Africa or Asia where Christian persecutions are still very common, that just wouldn't be true. The mission work I did was in Canada of all places. I know, not very riveting. I served with an organization called NET Ministries of Canada. NET focused on the New Evangelization: evangelizing the baptized. I served for two years with NET where I traveled the country putting on retreats and helping parishes start up youth groups of their own.

No, I wasn't faced with death or third world conditions every day, but the challenges came in ways that have helped me in literally every aspect of my life since then. These challenges were the kind that stretch you and make you grow up.

The growing pains came in two forms. The first was the physical challenges. Yes the -40° wasn't terribly fun, thanks Canada, but the temperature wasn't the hard part. Quite often we went with very little sleep.

Our average day consisted of waking up at 5 a.m. in order to either start the retreat in time or hit the road for our next 12 hour road trip. There are plenty of people who wake up at 5 without complaint, but the early mornings weren't the hard part. The challenging part was staying up until midnight or 1 a.m. the night before because you needed to spend time with your host family who took you into their home for the night that made the early mornings so rough. Take all this, add putting on retreats every day for kids, and multiply it by 10 months a year for 2 years and you'll get a sense of how tired we were on a daily basis.

The mental effort came not with putting on retreats and having to work with kids every day, that part was usually ok, but with your team. Anyone can relate to getting a little annoyed or irritated at someone you have to spend all day with at work or on a trip, and this was no exception for us. We traveled, worked, ate, and lived together for 10 months. The first month or so was ok for both my years because everyone was still in the whole "I don't know you so I can't let you know I'm mad at you stage". This quickly faded, however, after spending every moment together for a few weeks. Even missionaries are imperfect.

The amazing part of these two years for me was how much it forced me to grow as a person. If I had a problem with a team member I had to talk to them and work it out because our ministry could suffer if other people noticed that we were having a disagreement. We had to put aside our feelings and preferences and hash things out for the sake of our mission. Some people found this easy, but I, being the low-key people pleaser that I am, never got to that point. The fact that I didn't like conflict didn't matter though. All that mattered was spreading the Kingdom of Heaven and we knew we needed to work together in order to do that.

I think a lot of people have some period of their lives that forces them to grow, put their feelings aside, and get done what they need to get done. Unfortunately for some they have no prior experience of this and so, when it happens, tend to go into a defensive posture. Think of all of the kids who grow up getting A's and B's passed out to them for barely any work. They ran the race and got the participation trophy, even though they finished dead last. They grow up having everything handed to them and so never encounter any resistance, and without resistance, there can be no growth.

This is not just me psychoanalyzing people being spoiled. We see this in nature as well. Do you know how muscles grow bigger and stronger? The muscle fibers in whatever muscle you are working on are asked to perform some function, say performing a push up, and, in order to lift and lower your body, each of the individual fibers within the muscle must contract in order for your muscles to make your skeletal system move in the way you need it to. If the force asked for is more than that main muscle (or prime mover) is capable of producing, your brain

will recruit secondary muscles to help
get the job done. When your prime mover
muscle has exerted itself to a greater degree
than it has in the past you actually will find
thousands, if not millions, of microscopic rips
within the fibers (think of how you feel when
you are sore). So what does your body do?
It adapts. It repairs the damaged fibers and
makes them bigger and stronger than before,
so they don't tear under that weight again.

In a similar way that's how we
grow emotionally and mentally. We have
to be asked something of ourselves that
seems slightly beyond our abilities, strive
to accomplish it at the risk of failure, and
come out on the other side. Sometimes
we succeed and at other times we fail.
The result isn't what's important. The
important thing is the path you took.

You don't grow as an athlete at
tournaments and games. You grow at 5:00
a.m. when you are grinding it out at the gym
or on the field. You grow when it's 98° outside
and you sweat through the hour and a half

practice. The games and tournaments are simply where you put your growth to the test.

Growth isn't the ultimate purpose though. We don't want to grow for the sake of growing. We want to grow as people for the sake of serving both God and others. Everything is for the goal of being a sincere gift like we mentioned earlier. We don't seek mastery of our bodies for a six pack. The pursuit of mastery of our bodies is so, when we are asked to serve in some way, we have practiced commanding our bodies to do what it needs to do. We have trained ourselves how to set aside how we feel for the sake of attaining our goal and so we can get that cup of coffee for our tired spouse, or that bottle for our crying baby.

As silly as it might sound, I didn't believe people when they told me how hard it was to take care of a newborn. I knew it would have its challenges and that I would be more tired than usual, but I don't think I was quite ready for the beautiful struggle that it was. I don't think anyone can quite be prepared for being exhausted, waking up at 2 a.m. only to change yet another diaper that is filled with more matter than you think is possible to come out of someone so small and cute. Some nights you go through the motions and everything goes smoothly. Other nights the baby has a stuffy nose, so feeding is exceptionally difficult and you remember that diaper changing becomes a whole lot harder when the lights are off and you don't have your glasses on.

Have I lost my patience with my little girl and spouse at times? Unfortunately, yes. But I realized that my past experiences as a missionary, watching other parents, including my own, and all of the other seemingly unimportant moments of service, gave me both the tools and experience to grow as a husband and father. I've had years of little sleep as a missionary to help me cope with long nights, and I have been taught how to have an open and peaceful dialogue in order to avoid serious confrontations. My wife and I aren't perfect but we have never raised our voices at each other or our daughter. Why? Because we strive to conquer ourselves in order to not allow how we feel or what is happening *to* us to affect how we treat others. Like I mentioned earlier: self discipline isn't for yourself, it's for others. Getting angry and losing your temper can't be blamed on your temperament or personality. Someone might be more prone to *feeling* the emotion of anger because of their temperament, but *losing* your temper and taking it out on others is entirely your fault. The difference is in the choice. We can't stop the feeling, but whatever we do with it is on us and no one else.

You might be thinking "Well that's all fine and good but I've never been and will probably never be a full time missionary." But that isn't the point of the story. The load given to each of us is given as an opportunity to break out of our selfishness. The idea is simple: calculated exposure to adversity gives you the tools to overcome challenges in larger and larger amounts, helping you to build habits of sacrifice. Habits that help you and those around on the path to heaven. That only happens when we learn to encounter pain and not live our lives doing everything possible to avoid it.

Spiritual Challenge:

Take time today to meditate and pray on how you respond to discomfort. Do you become defensive? Do you lash out at those close to you? What about the times when it sneaks up on you and you aren't "ready" for it? Ask the Holy Spirit to guide you through this self examination.

Physical Challenge:

The next time someone annoys you, or you find yourself uncomfortable around someone, compliment them.

Theosis: Becoming God's Perfect Children

Ok, so we are about to enter into some deeper theological waters here. While this is not a theology book, it is important to remember that our ultimate goal is heaven. That's it. We aren't writing this book to make you the next super model or fitness elite. We want you to get to heaven and we believe that fitness is one of the essential elements to help you along the way, and this happens through something called *theosis*.

The reality of our divine adoption and how we enter into heaven as sons and daughters, is one that has been analyzed and discussed by theologians since St. Paul. This is important to stress in order to show that in no way are we stating anything new in this chapter. We will simply be restating truths that have been revealed to us through the scriptures and the tradition of the Church. The reason that this topic of divine adoption has been so widely discussed is because it is literally the way of salvation, and the foundation for Christianity. So yeah, kind of important. The Catechism, quoting St. Thomas Aquinas, puts it this way: "The only-begotten Son of God, wanting to make us sharers in his divinity, assumed our nature, so that he, made man, might make men gods" (CCC 460).

In the beginning of salvation history we are presented with the reality that Adam was created as a son of God. "So God created man in his own image, in the image of God he created him; male and female he created them" (Gen 1:27). At first this can appear as merely a metaphor for the creation of man, but Genesis 5 points us in a different direction. The author of Genesis begins chapter five by bringing our attention back to the beginning: "When God created man, he made him in the likeness of God. Male and female he created them, and he blessed them and named them Man when they were created" (Gen 5:1-2). With our attention now fixed on Adams origins the author then pivots. "When Adam had lived a hundred and thirty years, he became the father of a son in his *own likeness, after his image*, and named him Seth" (Gen 5:3). The repetition of the words "likeness" and "image" are intentional. If "image" and "likeness" are used with Adam's literal son Seth, then we are supposed to take that to mean that Adam, in some mysterious way, is God's son.

This does not mean that this happened naturally. The Bible can *literally* say something without meaning it happened *naturally.* What made Adam the son of God wasn't that God engendered Adam's human nature, for God is pure spirit and therefore could not have given anything physical. What made Adam a son had to be something immaterial. What are the only 3 immaterial things that Adam possessed? His intellect, will, and grace.

Long story short, every human has the first two (intellect & will) naturally, that's what separates us from animals. So we are left with the last option that made Adam a literal son of God: grace. God's very essence dwelling in Adam's soul. That is what made original sin so devastating. It's not that Adam was given a stain that he would later pass on to his offspring, and later us. Rather, he lost the true presence of God that made him a literal son. And he couldn't give what he didn't have, so from that point on the rest of humanity would be left with this hole in our hearts until Christ came and offered us adoption through baptism. "But now that faith has come, we are no longer under a custodian; for in Christ Jesus you are all sons of God, through faith. For as many of you as were baptized into Christ have put on Christ" (Gal 3:25-27).

Baptism is only the beginning point though. Yes, we are made sons and daughters but here's the catch: heaven is where perfectly loving children dwell with their perfectly loving God and Father, and you and I don't love perfectly, not yet anyway. That is where all of this ties into fitness. Baptism is the starting point. Theosis is the journey *and* the goal. Fitness is just one of the ways to practice fasting and asceticism (more on this in the next chapter) in order to conform our hearts of stone into hearts of flesh (2 Corinthians 3) that can love God and others perfectly.

Think we are setting the bar too high? That Jesus is simply asking you to be "nice" and that heaven will magically drop into your lap? Maybe you read the Sermon on the Mount (Matthew 5-7) that way, but it is hard to argue with Jesus when he says "Be perfect, as your Heavenly Father is perfect" (Mt 5:48). The call to perfection is the call to theosis. God's power and inner life dwelling in us empowers us to stretch beyond mere human capability to reach this impossibly high bar.

If you are thinking of quitting before you start because this all sounds a bit too difficult, then you're looking at the problem backwards. You would be right in saying that you can't do it on your own because it's literally impossible without the Holy Spirit. God's not asking anything of us that he's not prepared to give us everything we need to accomplish. He extends his hand, asks us to trust, and shows us each next step one at a time. We don't have to have the whole track to our perfection clearly outlined with milestones and timestamps, we just need to know whether our next step is left or right. When you're driving at night, you can't see the whole road – you can really only see 30 feet in front of you – but you can get all the way to your destination that way.

God is offering us something pretty radical, something impossible by human standards. The scriptures, the sacraments, and his Church are the primary channels through which he supplies the means and the nourishment on our journey but we're not without responsibility in this relationship. He calls, we answer. It's worth asking ourselves "How am I responding to that call right now?". Maybe you're even at the place of needing to ask "Do I hear or acknowledge his call at all?". This book is all about our response. We're here to help you start forming the habits that will build you up to answer that call every day. We're here to give you an appreciation for asceticism.

Spiritual Challenge:

Pray through the Sermon on the Mount (Matthew 5-7) this week. Ask God where he's asking you to start your journey of theosis.

Physical Challenge:

When is the last time you hit a mile run/power walk hard? This week, do a mile as fast as you can. Whether you power walk, jog or run, that doesn't matter. Write down the time and set a goal of beating that time next month.

OVERCOMING SELF

The Art of Fasting

An idea that we cannot stress enough is that we are not reinventing the wheel or putting words in Jesus' mouth when we talk about faith and fitness. St. Paul uses olympian runners as an analogy of the faith:

> *Do you not know that in a race all the runners compete, but only one receives the prize? So run that you may obtain it. Every athlete exercises self-control in all things. They do it to receive a perishable wreath, but we an imperishable. Well, I do not run aimlessly, I do not box as one beating the air; but I pommel my body and subdue it, lest after preaching to others I myself should be disqualified (1 Cor 9:24-27)*

This analogy is amazing because it gives us three key characteristics of those who take the spiritual journey seriously. The first comes from Aristotle's idea that the goal is always the first in thought and the last in attaining. Before you set out to do anything, you have a goal in mind. Someone doesn't enter a tournament simply because they want to, but to win.

Once the runners have their goal in mind (to win) they then train in order that they are prepared to attain it. They wake up before sunrise, eat certain foods, avoid other foods they might like, go to bed at a good time, and train for hours, all to be able to compete well.

Lastly, they "run as to obtain it (the prize)". Once they begin the race they leave nothing in the tank. They push themselves and give 100% until they reach the finish line.

Do we do the same?

What St. Paul is talking about here is called asceticism. Mathias Nygaard breaks down this word for us: "The term 'asceticism' stems from the Greek word for 'training' or 'exercising' (ἄσκησις, *askēsis*). In classical Greek, this term is often used to describe people such as athletes or soldiers who engage in certain exercises to attain a goal. With time, the term 'ascetic' came to denote a person who practices the virtues"

Asceticism falls under the umbrella of fasting. This isn't just some optional practice for Christians to separate the "hard core" Catholics from the casual ones, or something that we only do during Lent and Advent. Fasting is something Jesus *assumes* his disciples are already doing.

> *And when you fast, do not look dismal, like the hypocrites, for they disfigure their faces that their fasting may be seen by men. Truly, I say to you, they have received their reward. But when you fast, anoint your head and wash your face, that your fasting may not be seen by men but by your Father who is in secret; and your Father who sees in secret will reward you (Mt 6:16–18).*

Notice that Jesus did not say "if" you fast, but "when you fast". Jesus is doing the same thing here that he does in the rest of the Sermon on the Mount, where this text comes from. He is taking the standard spiritual ideal and practice and elevating it into the higher plane of authentic Christian love. Fasting had been practiced by the Israelites for centuries, but the Jews of Jesus' day had turned it into a competition rather than a practice of love and dying to self for the glory of God.

In today's fitness culture we see people practicing natural asceticism and fasting all the time. Especially in the fitness industry, we have seen the intermittent fasting trend take off for various health reasons or to lose weight. People practice this natural asceticism by working out or avoiding junk food, but when you ask someone to fast or practice asceticism for God all of the sudden it becomes this unbearable ideal that is simply unrealistic. This reaction shows us that we are falling into the idolatry of the body.

There are two extremes that we must do our very best to avoid when approaching fitness and asceticism: idolatry and platonism. Too many people who focus on physical fitness turn their bodies into idols. Sound extreme? Think of all of the people who make literally every decision around their diet and workout schedule. If they eat one thing "wrong" or don't get all their steps in, they lose their peace. They spend hours over the course of a week, or a day, looking at themselves in the mirror either praising or hating themselves. Their physical appearance turns into the marker of their worth and success.

The other side of this coin is practical platonism. Plato believed that our souls were trapped in our bodies and were trying to "escape". This made the body, and everything physical, an evil because it hindered the soul, the true person, from being where it was meant to be. While most of us don't have this extreme view, a lot of well intentioned Christians spend their spiritual journey neglecting their body. Sometimes they have this false idea that their soul is not going to be affected. This can take shape in a lot of ways, like: eating unhealthy foods all of the time, drinking too much, neglecting physical activity, or even not eating enough (over-fasting) for the sake of being "spiritual". Don't get me wrong, like we have been talking about, fasting is a beautiful practice that truly helps you grow in the spiritual life. It is important to remember that most of the extreme fasts that we read about from the saints were approved by their spiritual directors, and that I am primarily addressing lay people here, not cloistered nuns or hermits. The mistake that some lay people make is attempting a fast that prevents them from fulfilling their daily duties, which differ greatly from those of nuns and hermits. They become so tired and lethargic that they end up sinning in a different way because they lack the necessary energy.

It took a priest in a confessional to point out this mistake to me. When my wife and I were dating we decided to do a fast during Lent where we would only eat bread and water every Wednesday and Friday. We found that Wednesday's weren't bad but Friday's were extremely difficult. After a few weeks I noticed that I was being short and snarky with her on Friday's, and that I was having a hard time being joyful on the days I was fasting. I mentioned this during confession one day and what the priest said shook me out of my spiritual pride. "You know fasting isn't supposed to make you a jerk, right?"

His words were incredibly humbling because it was in that conversation that he told me that this fast might be too extreme for me and I wasn't ready for it. He instructed us to get rid of the Wednesday fast and only do it on Fridays. Sure enough, I stopped being a jerk on my fast days and found that I was entering deeper into my prayer with both joy and love.

So what's the middle ground here? If one extreme is idolatry of the body and the other side is practical platonism, then the virtue is somewhere in the middle. Fortunately that's exactly where the Church desires us to be. We ought to train our bodies in order to keep us healthy, fit, and grow in virtue. We should use this training as a springboard to help us grow in our faith. This is self mastery for the sake of service. The middle ground is what St. John Paul II found in *Gaudium et Spes*: "man, who is the only creature on earth which God willed for itself, cannot fully find himself except through a sincere gift of himself."

Is this easy? Of course not. Nothing amazing ever is.

Spiritual Challenge:

Pick a day this week to not watch TV, movies, or sports for the whole day. Stay away from social media and your phone. Fill this time with spiritual reading, prayer, or with quality time with a friend or family member.

Physical Challenge:

Fast this Friday. Abstain from eating meat and only have 1 normal meal and 2 snacks that don't equal a full meal. If you want to add an element of difficulty, only drink 1 black coffee and water that day. Don't do it on the same day as the spiritual challenge above.

"The life of a Christian is nothing but a perpetual struggle against self; there is no flowering of the soul to the beauty of its perfection except at the price of pain"
- Padre Pio

The Spirituality of Mortification

One of my favorite movies is the Princess Bride. Not a hard thing to imagine, I'd say it's on a lot of peoples' Top 10 lists. But one line that strikes me every time I hear it is when Princess Buttercup, distraught, protests to Wesley that he mocks her pain, to which he fiercely replies:

"Life is pain, princess! Anyone who says otherwise is selling something"

What a line! And one that I must confess I didn't immediately love. In fact, the first time I heard that line spoken I balked. What was he talking about? There are plenty of enjoyable parts of life. I suspect there was a part of me that also didn't *want* that to be true. After all, what life is worth living if it's defined by pain? But I couldn't shake the feeling that there was some way in which what he was saying was actually true – and that scared me! However, God has slowly and mercifully led me on a journey by which I have come to see the beauty (and truth) of Wesley's maxim. To see the joy on the other side of pain.

From our first moments outside the womb, the presence of pain is as near to us as our breath. In fact, it is part of what defines our experience of life. No one can avoid it. At some point illness, heartbreak, injury, loneliness, age, seperation, and conflict wrap their stony claws on our innocence. There are physical pains, emotional pains, spiritual pains. Pains inflicted on us by others and those that seem to come by misfortune. Quick, sharp pains and long, enduring pains. The pains that we experience and the pain of seeing those we love suffer. From the simplest daily frustrations to the diseases that inflict lifelong debilitations, a thread of *struggle* characterizes the human experience.

How could you look at life and say that it's *not* pain.

There is a spectrum of intensity to the pains that I listed but there is not a single day that passes where we don't experience pain or discomfort on some level. It's worth mentioning that this is the experience of so many of us in the first world but that there are countless individuals around the globe whose daily sufferings are far more intense than we'll ever know.

To try to run from this reality is to run from life, and that's not an easy statement to make. The only way I've found to bear this unbearable truth (and the way typified by Christ) is to *lean into* the pain and force it to work for your good. To become pain's master and invite the transforming power of grace into those dark realities.

The pains of life are things we endure, they are passive sufferings. We don't exercise any level of control over whether they come to us or not. But there are sufferings that we do control and pains that we willingly endure. Our mentality has an immense influence on the way in which we bear our pains and adopting an attitude of acceptance performs the ironic function of actually lessening the burden. On a spiritual level this is conforming our will to the Will of God; surrendering to Divine Providence.

Mortifications are the practice that we give ourselves in learning to bear pain well. They are the little practices that prepare us for the playoffs of life. To *mortify* is to put to death. The mortifications we adopt bring focus and clarity by lessening our interior dependence on anything that may distract us from our ultimate goal.

Exercise is a type of mortification. We intentionally place ourselves in positions where we encounter pain for an extended period of time in order to grow. Someone who has progressed in the spiritual life, and in their fitness journey, is someone who has learned to encounter this specific pain and let it transform them.

Spiritual Challenge:

What is your disposition toward fasting and mortification? Is it one of fear or desire? Is it a source of pride? Or does it help you cleanse your soul of false attachments? Offer your mortifications to God through Mary. Ask her help in adding, subtracting, or adjusting your bodily disciplines to most fittingly love and serve God and neighbor. Let her rearrange the array of your offering like the roses in Juan Diego' tilma

Physical Challenge:

Go for a run this week. This is not supposed to be a casual jog, find that point of pain and lean into it. Hold on to it for as long as you can, then try to do it a little longer the next time around.

Jesus' Pain

Jesus Christ is the model *par excellence* of using the touchpoints of pain, resistance, weakness, and outright evil as the channel through which God renews creation. As St. Paul says,

"My grace is sufficient for you, for power is made perfect in weakness." So, I will boast all the more gladly of my weaknesses, so that the power of Christ may dwell in me." (2 Cor 12:9).

Of the punishments incurred at the Fall, death was the fiercest. But by Christ, the instrument of our downfall becomes the sure path to glory. He gives explicit instructions that our daily task is to shoulder that burden and march confidently toward our death. It's a startling cosmic irony that death is no longer a cliff that we fall off of but a door that we pass through.

This irony didn't just suddenly

manifest at the resurrection, though. God
has always been at work transforming
the creation that continues to stray
from him. The incarnation means that
that transformation is now possible
in the deepest parts of our being.

If we are open to the possibility that
even the worst situations may in time bear
some good, then all of life is joy and every
affliction is bearable. If we don't believe that
radical change can occur (in ourselves or
in others) and see only momentary pain,
then no victory will be sufficient and peace
will *never* find a home in our hearts.

All of creation - and most
importantly all of mankind - are being
kneaded under the gentle and perfectly
wise hands of the Father, transforming
what is not like Him into that which is.

In the symphony that is the created
world, He takes every sour note through
which we try to usurp the orchestration
and he adjusts the melody so that it's not

a mistake but the start of a new theme.

Creation is hard. Destruction is easy. Making something again after it has been destroyed is supremely difficult and impossible for the impatient. But God's own response to evil and destruction from the very start has been the humble glory of re-creation. To use the malefactions that plague every good thing he created as opportunities to bring about even more splendid realities than had previously been. To use free will gone wrong in a million situations as the inaugurations of an avalanche of blessings means that we say with St. Ambrose and the rest of the church, "Felix culpa!", O, happy fault, that in the face of disobedience and tyranny we are brought, even still, to greater joys.

Nothing God made is ever truly lost. No effort in vain. No element unused. No space left void. At the end of time God will take stock of all that he once put into the world and show that he lost nothing along the way. As Isaiah says of the Lord: "so shall my word be that goes out from my mouth; it shall not return to me empty" (Is 55:11). Each attempt at destruction was surmounted by his ingenious and infinite creativity, so that no things are unmade but all things are made new.

Each encounter we have with pain is our small taste of the 'undoing' which nips at our heels and has since our first steps on this earth. Each encounter is our opportunity to hand things over to life-giving transformation. Each encounter with pain should be our joy because it is our chance to see not just what *is* but what *could be*. It's a chance for things to improve in ways they never could before.

Since our Savior has chosen not to eliminate but to transmute darkness, we must follow his example. All in all, it does us the most good to make friends with the place where it hurts because if we can be assured of one thing, it's that we'll be seeing each other again.

Spiritual Challenge:

*Pray through one of the Passion Narratives
(Mt 26:30-27:66, Mk 14:26-15:47,
Lk 22:39-23:56, Jn 18:1-19:42)*

Physical Challenge:

*Find a hill near you. If you don't have
one, set a treadmill incline up as high as
it can go. Do 12 sprints up the hill (or 12
30-second sprints on the treadmill) and
offer each one for someone you love.*

So, what does all this have to do with working out?

*The moral virtues grow through education,
deliberate acts, and perseverance in struggle.
Divine grace purifies and elevates them.*
- CCC 1839

As an activity characterized by struggle, exercise turns the gym (or track, or pool, or bike - pick your arena) into a place where our surrender to providence is practiced, our spiritual endurance is formed, and where we overcome ourselves for the sake of something greater. Placing your "why" as the object of whatever difficulty you've elected for the day gives purpose, energy, and direction to what would otherwise be flailing your arms around.

Firstly, as we'll mention over and over in this book: as creatures made for self-gift, it's fundamental to our nature and part of our immortal destiny to sacrifice. Self-possession precedes self-gift – you can't give what you don't have – and in practicing mortifications we routinely assert the dominance of our will and establish the habits that break down our slavery to impulse.

Secondly, voluntary suffering is a way to prepare our wills to receive every suffering we will face. The acknowledgement of struggle as one of the inescapable realities of life and the acceptance that somewhere in the mind of God that struggle is permissible and, in fact, the *best possible* road disposes the soul for the inevitable adversities that it encounters. It provides hope in difficulty and – even more deeply – becomes a way that we come to know the heart of the Creator.

Thirdly, the stewardship of our bodies is an act of gratitude to God and honors the marvel he has wrought in the human form. It seems obvious here to reference the parable of the talents (Matt 25:14-30) and the exceedingly Catholic notion of stewardship by which we acknowledge everything in our possession as gifts to be not only cared for but cultivated. Seeds without water don't grow. Humanity crowns creation with every part of their being and the Genesis account makes - with resounding clarity - the case for man as a gardener; one of whose primary functions is the care and cultivation of the created world. To exempt our bodies from that care is to neglect that which is the most precious to Our Lord.

Jesus was not broken for the humpback whale, God did not die on calvary for the sake of the Grand Canyon or the Amazon rainforest, he gave himself over to unimaginable tortures in order to achieve the most intimate, familiar, and bodily communion with the creatures that he did not see fit to weather eternity without.

Spiritual Challenge:

What is your initial emotional reaction when you think about working out, or going to the gym? Why do you think you react the way you do? Bring that to God and talk with him about it.

Physical Challenge:

Limit your consumption of either alcohol or junk food by half (at least) this week.

Pillar Three

GROWING THE GIFT

The Soil & Fruit of the Catholic Fitness Journey

Everything is a gift. Everything. While we are on this journey towards making our lives gifts of self in order that we may truly find ourselves through fitness, we can't forget that we can only cooperate with the initial gifts of grace and life that God has given us. We recognize these graces more when we are in constant dialogue with the gift giver through prayer. Prayer is the soil upon which all our progress lies. It is where we draw our nourishment and strength from him who is the way, truth, and life (Jn 14:6). The amazing thing about authentic Catholic prayer is that it is not complicated. As St. Therese of Lisieux states, "For me, prayer is a surge of the heart; it is a simple look turned toward heaven, it is a cry of recognition and of love, embracing both trial and joy." Yet, just because something isn't complicated doesn't mean it's easy.

I would argue that most well-intentioned Catholics pray by at least raising a quick thought or thanksgiving to God every day. While this is a good start, it's not enough. Prayer is a relationship. It is not something that "helps" your relationship with God, prayer *is* the relationship (CCC 2565). If you only spoke to your spouse, or best friends, for 1 or 2 seconds a day, what would the relationship look like in 5, 10, or 20 years? Odds are, not very good. Sure, you would have some familiarity with them, but you wouldn't be able to tell me the depth of their heart-- their fears, struggles, hopes, and joys. The challenge for us is to make prayer an intentional part of our day.

One of the many benefits my wife and I gained from our marriage prep course was the idea of "dating your spouse". This is a great thing to do to keep a marriage fresh and engaged. We should also take this approach to our relationship with God. Let me explain.

The idea behind dating your spouse

is to intentionally set aside a period of time every week in order to have quality time with each other; to check in, reconnect, and lean on each other for support through life. The same should happen with God. We should intentionally set aside a period of time every day in order to reconnect with the God who loves us. This happens best in silence.

Have you ever tried to listen to your spouse's heartbeat? My wife loves to lay her head on my chest before bed and just listen to mine. It calms her down and she finds that it is a simple way to be physically intimate without having to do anything but be silent.

This is the goal of prayer: to hear the heartbeat of Jesus. Our desire should be to imitate St. John who laid on Jesus' breast at the last supper (Jn 13:23). It is there that we will find our repose and our strength.

If prayer is the soil then what is the fruit? The answer: virtue. "A virtue is an *habitual* and *firm* disposition to do the good. It allows the person not only to perform good acts, but *to give the best of himself*. The virtuous person tends toward the good with all his sensory and spiritual powers; he pursues the good and chooses it in *concrete actions*" (CCC 1803; emphasis added). A lot can be said about virtues and many books have been written - literally since Aristotle - on the subject. Let's simply break down the above text to show how virtue is the fruit of the Catholic fitness lifestyle.

Firstly, virtues are "habitual and firm dispositions". That means that you don't magically become virtuous the moment you do one good thing. Anyone can be forced to do a good thing and never do it again. Think about how long it takes to teach children good manners and to be polite. You start from the time that they can actually comprehend the do's and don'ts. Then, you continue to remind them, and force (or bribe them when necessary) until they learn the "habit" of being polite. The hope is that one day they even like being polite to others. They acquire the *virtue* or "politeness" when they do it habitually and they enjoy doing it.

Second, "It allows the person not only to perform good acts, but *to give the best of himself*". For your life to be a "sincere gift of self" you must have virtue because that's what empowers you to give your best, not just your leftovers. It is the virtuous person who is able to master himself and order his life towards serving others, resisting temptation, and enjoy the life that Christ calls us to live in the Sermon on the Mount (Matt 5-7).

Thirdly, the virtuous person "pursues the good and chooses it in *concrete actions*". This isn't some theoretical idea or abstract concept. If you are virtuous you *will* do good deeds. You won't be able to help yourself! That is why just "being nice" to people won't cut it. You have to serve them. Your entire self, body, mind and soul, must become a gift to them. That is what makes virtue tricky. In order to acquire it, you must have it in seed form to even think about doing it, and in order to grow in it, you must do it.

Prayer is how we hear the heart of Jesus and virtue is how we live out what we hear. St. Gregory of Nyssa put it this way: "The goal of a virtuous life is to become like God." Theosis is once again at the heart of the message here. The Catholic fitness lifestyle is theosis of the whole person. Prayer is the soil and virtue is the fruit. Your life is the tree. When you first start out, you will look a bit pitiful and will get tossed around by the wind and rain. But if you stick to it – if you really press into Jesus – your roots will get deeper and you will be able to draw even more grace from the soil of prayer, and eventually you will bear such amazing fruit that others will come to you for nourishment and strength.

Spiritual Challenge:

*Decide on a time to set aside every day
for personal prayer. Set a reminder
if you need to. Tell someone so they
can keep you accountable.*

Physical Challenge:

*Read the Catechism of the Catholic Church's
section on Virtue (CCC 1803-1845). Find
a virtue you want to work on and take
practical actions to grow in this virtue.*

Health and Service to Others

There are practical reasons for exercise that draw meaning from it's spiritual components but are very grounded in our day-to-day, human experiences.

Fitness isn't a very intellectual activity. We've outlined a good amount of the rationale, the logical backdrop for sanctifying it as a practice, but exercise is primarily physical. This is one of the reasons that we believe it is so potent as a proto-spiritual springboard.

Not everyone can discuss philosophy or theology at the same level, in fact many find it so difficult they never try. Everyone can understand what it is to feel strong, though. They can understand when something hurts and are capable of finding that place within themselves where they find the strength to push through a difficult activity. The discipline that fitness requires is a perfect analogue to the discipline of prayer. Beyond that it is also a great accent to those already adept in prayer as it humanizes and grounds invisible realities in our physical experiences .

The word "fitness" is telling and reiterates the fruits of virtue that stem from its tree. Something that is fit is acceptable. *Someone* who is fit is prepared to serve competently. A willing heart is nothing if a person is unable to physically carry out their intentions. Finding the place within ourselves that desires to give (that place in our hearts sourced in the divine) is one piece of a two-part puzzle. Without action our intentions to be of service are vanity. Conversely, service without love is a different kind of vanity. The two must dwell together.

We receive physical benefits in using and stretching our bodies - the natural consequences of exercise - and those benefits become gifts to others.

There are the personal benefits of

health, mobility, and longevity. Ironic as it may be, willfully seeking out (an albeit moderately) painful activity we condition and prepare our bodies for a *less painful* existence. The lack of self-concern that arises from our bodily systems operating well disposes our availability to others and gives us the opportunity to ponder ways that we can minister to those around us (if we choose to do so -- there are those who use their health as an opportunity to further their self-indulgence and vanity, like we mentioned earlier).

Communally, our health is also the way that we become available to those that God has placed in our lives (firstly our family and then our neighbors and community). Being able to respond to the manifold physical needs encountered in the human experience is an incredible gift that can only be given through the stewardship of our bodies and our strength.

We respond in this way when a friend needs help moving and we lend a hand.

We support our families when our health doesn't prevent us from playing with our children or grandchildren; when our diet replenishes our energy and properly fuels us. We give a gift to our children in taking such care of our bodies so as to see them and their children grow up and get married. We support our community by volunteering ourselves, our hands, our backs to moments of community togetherness or the care and nursing of the sick and elderly.

Overcoming the temptation to view exercise and fitness as "time spent on self" and allowing the time that you spend on yourself to refine and energize you builds a strong foundation for increasing the capacity of what you are able to give as your gift. I'm reminded of the widow in Mark's gospel who gave of everything she had (Mk 12:41) and the little drummer boy from the popular christmas song, who, though poor, gave of all that they had with their whole hearts. How pleased the Father was with their gifts!

A heart full of love desires to give

more and more; to shower the object of affection with every conceivable good thing so that even in scarcity the heart sacrifices what little belongs to them for the sake of the other. But even after giving, the heart still loves. Even after sacrificing all the heart sees that *all* is never enough. The widow, after giving her last pennies, wishes she could have given ten hundred pennies. Imagine the little drummer boy, after expending his performance, would be filled with such fire to go back to his home and practice his drumming and become so advanced that he could gather the most talented musicians he knew and marshall a spectacular performance, fit for royalty, and play that song again and again for the pleasure of the Lord. Nothing can exhaust that burning flame of gift in love because love *is* self-gift and love is eternal. *Deus caritas est.* God is love.

For this reason the fullness of heart mentioned above flows from a deep relationship with the Father through prayer and manifests in a desire to make of oneself a continually more perfect offering. To take our talents (Mt 25:13-40) and multiply them not for our own benefit (though that accompanies one's gift as a consequence) but to give them to the object of our love, the One who is most deserving, and to give them to Him through his children. This is all part of the journey to self-gift.

Spiritual Challenge:

Pray through Matthew 5. Think of someone you wouldn't usually help out and find some way of serving them.

Physical Challenge:

Set a fitness goal that you want to hit three months from now. Then write down why you want to hit that goal and who it will serve.

Pillar Four

THE GIFT IN YOUR LIFE

The Practical Ascetic

We've used the word a few times, but 'ascetic' isn't something you hear thrown around too much these days. It's a word that comes to us through the wisdom and tradition of the church that – despite it's scary sound – is actually something deep, meaningful, and not at all impossible for the average modern Catholic (see *The Art of Fasting* chapter for definition).

Simply put, it's a concentrated daily approach to mastering our impulses and stewarding our bodies in the ultimate effort to get ourselves and our loved ones to heaven.

So, what does that mean?

What we're hoping to begin with this book is a *movement*. A modern swelling of the faithful – especially the laity – in an increased effort to holiness and sanctity through our ordinary lives.

Almost all of us will not be called to grand acts of martyrdom but we are each called (much more importantly) to love our neighbor. We're looking to start a revitalization among this generation of those who take seriously the "universal call to holiness". There is not one person exempted from the glory, expressions, and demands of humanity's divine destiny.

What that looks like in each individual life varies wildly. In my life right now the road to sanctity is having patience with slow old ladies who drive 20 miles under the speed limit with their left blinker on. It's forgiving my in-laws when their cat pees on my couch (again!). It's resisting the urge to karate chop the clueless old man who just asked my highly emotional pregnant wife if she's having twins (she's not, by the way).

What we're talking about is a thousand small, sanctifying acts that slowly but surely bring a greater and greater degree of clarity to the kingdom of Heaven in the domain of our lives. Which, by the way, is not to say they are *easier*, just *better*.

An ascetic, in our context, is someone who mounts the challenge of self-mastery every single day and not only endures the chastisements of God but seeks to apply them to himself. A practical ascetic, to us, is really just a Christian; because that's where we believe the Gospel leads.

Our world is crowded with an unbelievable amount of noise. We are faced with the daily temptations to succumb to distraction, indulge our every desire, and build an altar to our ego. But the Christian faith is countercultural, and it always will be. To follow Christ is a *struggle*. Our Lord is not confusing at all on the topic and calls every day a cross!

The ascetic kisses the cross.

The ascetic recalls the words of the Good Shepherd who says "my yoke is easy and my burden is light" (Mt 11:28). As we mentioned in the section about pain, Christians are blessed with knowledge

of the paradoxical truth that the path
beyond pain leads through it and that
our God is a god of persistent goodness
who brings light out of dark, healing out
of tragedy, good out of evil, and life out of
death. We're not fanatics or masochists
but brothers and sisters who have been
wounded and have seen our Healer be
wounded and surmount that wound.

The ascetic strives to live more deeply
through a focus beyond the immediate; to
live more happily through a focus on *true*
love and a relationship with the Prime Lover.

The practical ascetic is able to
give because they possess and what
they possess they have through the daily
discipline of self-mastery. Exercise is
one important way that that mastery is
gained but it is only part of a more complex
disposition to give and receive love based
on a reception of the call to live a holy life.

Tangible Ascetical Habits

While we can't tell you exactly what *you* need to do in order to become a gift of self to others; we do want to impart a few practical things that we find very useful in our own lives when it comes to learning to be a gift to others. While extreme fasts and things like Exodus 90 can be hugely beneficial as a jump start, we desire that everyone instill habits of virtuous practices, not simply periods of time for them.

1. Start your day at 6:00am (or earlier if need be)

- When most people are told to start praying, or start working out, their first defensive move tends to be the legendary phrase "I just don't have the time". These people might very well be busy with work and kids, but I would also like to see how many hours a day they are on their cell phones, social media, or watching tv. By waking up early enough to have a cup of coffee with Jesus and hit the gym we are giving ourselves the time we need to grow every day.

- By starting your day at 6:00am you can also dive into the liturgy of the hours that are traditionally begun at 6:00am with Morning Prayer

2. Personal Prayer/Workout Combo

- This is where I think a lot of people vary. Personally, I like to start my mornings a little slower and have my cup of coffee with Jesus before I go workout. This pattern might work for you, or maybe you need to get the blood pumping before you can even think about sitting for 20-30 minutes without being tempted to fall back asleep. I think that both are good and, as long as they are both happening, can bear tremendous fruit.

- "According to St. Bonaventure, the morning and the evening are the two parts of the day which, ordinarily speaking, are the fittest for meditation. But, according to St. Gregory of Nyssa, the morning is the most seasonable time for prayer, because says the Saint, when prayer precedes business, sin will not find entrance into the soul. And the Venerable Father Charles Carafa, founder of the Congregation of the Pious Workers, used to say that a fervent act of love, made in the morning during meditation, is sufficient to maintain the soul in fervor during the entire day." - St. Alphonsis Ligouri

- A simple acronym that might help you structure your prayer is "P.L.A.D." (Praise, Listen, Ask, Dedicate)

- If you have never worked out before, getting to the gym for the first time can be intimidating. This is when finding a workout buddy or signing up for a fitness class can really come in handy.

We need accountability to ensure that we don't miss a workout. Decide on a number of times to workout every week (2 days a week is maintenance, 3 days is progress) and tell someone. Have them hold you accountable.

3. Fridays are Days of Penance

- Most modern Catholics tend to forget (or choose to ignore) the fact that Fridays throughout the *entire year* are considered penitential days (Canon 1250). Traditionally this has looked like giving up meat on Fridays but Canon 1253 has given the local Bishops the authority to make exceptions by means of substitution, if need be. Most of us tend to forget the substitution part. Giving up meat one day a week is a pretty easy way to make Friday's Penitential in honor of the Lord's Passion. But if this is not an option for you, find another way to honor Fridays throughout the entire year.

4. Serve Others

- Virtue, and developing virtue, is a bit weird if you think about it. Why? Because in order to grow in virtue, you must already possess it in some way. If you want to grow in bravery, you must practice being brave, but your desire and eventual brave action means that you already possess bravery in some capacity, no matter how small. We are striving to find ourselves through a sincere gift of self. This will require us to give of ourselves through service, which is why we practice everything written above. This "virtue seed", if we can call it that, has hopefully been planted and/or nourished in you from what you have read so far. Find small and big ways throughout your day (at work, home, or in your community) to serve those around you. Whether that's a greater degree of obedience to those with legitimate authority over you (parents, bosses, etc.), going out of your way to help those you've avoided in the past or whose company you dislike, or refraining from harsh or critical words there are a myriad of ways to increase every virtue through small steps. Ask the Lord for guidance and to reveal those opportunities to you while being open to whatever they may be.

Never Quit Early

One of the easiest things you can ever do, at least physically, is quit something. What does it require of you? Literally nothing except to stop moving. That's it. Simply stop moving, or stop showing up, and you will have accomplished your goal. That is why quitting is so tempting for us any time we reach that point of discomfort and potential pain, because it can be accomplished instantly and the reward is the immediate cessation of pain.

Like I mentioned way back in chapter 1, I grew up playing sports. What I didn't mention was my experience with baseball. For starters, I was never terribly good at it. I was that kid you see in the outfield picking weeds and playing with his glove. I also got hit with the ball one too many times (or 4 too many) when it would catch a divet in the ground or from a bad pitch, which didn't make me overly enthusiastic to play a game that would potentially hurt.

I remember the way my parents, who were huge baseball fans, handled the situation the first time I told them I didn't want to play any more. They didn't react one way or the other. They simply asked me why I didn't want to play. My answer? Because it hurts and it's hard. And here is where my parents did one of the best things any parent can ever do. They told me that those weren't good enough reasons to quit something and that I should play again next season. At first I was pretty annoyed. Why should I have to play a game that I don't think is fun any more? Don't they see I don't enjoy it? Of course they did, but they also saw a chance to build character in me by having me not quit something out of fear of discomfort.

The next season started shortly after and nothing had changed. I was still not very good and was timid around the ball. There was something that did change, though. I started getting really good at tennis.

I found a lot of joy in tennis and I was genuinely good at it. So, when that season of baseball ended I went up to my parents and told them I didn't want to play any more. They once again asked me why, but this time my response was different. I wanted to quit, not for the sake of ending discomfort, but in order to focus more of my time and energy on tennis. I wasn't saying "no" to baseball because it wasn't fun and was uncomfortable, instead I was saying "yes" to tennis. This was finally a good enough answer for my parents, and I am so thankful that they taught me this lesson when I was still young. The only fruit that quitting because something is uncomfortable or "not fun" will produce is that of weakness, idleness, and apathy.

We have to be careful not to interpret this as saying that it is *never* ok to stop something. There is a big difference between stopping and quitting. Stopping implies thought and deliberate decision making. Quitting is reactionary.

Throughout this book you have been presented with ideas that might have challenged you - at least that has been our hope. The thrust of our culture's messaging is to take the path of least resistance and glorify self-indulgence, whether that is through sexual pleasure, food, social acceptance, money, power, or fame. What we propose is fighting that culture of apathy, mediocrity, and indulgence, to empty yourself out in service of others.

We are asking you to be like St. Sebastian. Now some people know that St. Sebastian was shot with arrows by Roman soldiers after Emperor Diocletian found out that he was a Christian. While being shot with arrows for your faith is an astounding feat of faith, this is not what is most fascinating about his story. Sebastian knew Diocletian because he was a soldier of the guard that was assigned to protect him. After being betrayed by the man he swore to protect, shot with arrows, and left for dead, Sebastian was nursed back to health and did what very few of us could or would do: he returned to the Emperor to preach to him. Knowing that he would most likely be put to death again, he risked everything for a chance to save the Emperor's soul. After all, he had sworn to protect him, and for Sebastian, that meant more than making sure he didn't get physically hurt. St. Sebastian failed to convert Diocletian, however, and he was finally beaten to death with clubs and his body was tossed into a sewer.

While most of us are not going to be beaten or shot with arrows any time soon, what we need to imitate is St. Sebastian's willingness to die to himself over and over again. He had a reason for this: his "why" was the love of Jesus Christ and his love for the Emperor. He was willing to die for the slightest chance that he might convert the great persecutor of Christians.

Your "why" is what is going to help you not quit. Your "why" is what is going to give you the motivation to wake up early and pray and go to the gym. Hopefully at this point you have your "why", the primary reason you want to find yourself through a sincere gift of self by means of an authentically Catholic fitness journey. It won't be easy, but it will be worth it. It's now time for you to stop making excuses, to lace up those sneaks and get to work. Buy that gym membership, set that alarm early, pray, fast, and get to work.

Remember this is a marathon, not a sprint. We aren't looking for a quick 6-pack and chiseled arms, we are striving for sanctity. We are dying to ourselves for the sake of others. Not everyone is meant for the same level of exercise, but everyone is called to give more of themselves. That begins with our bodies and chances are, if you've made it this far in the book, you have a sense that the gym has a place in your life.

This book isn't supposed to give you all of the answers, it's supposed to get you up off your butt and after your better self. We're praying for each and every one of you.

Are you in for the journey?

continue your journey at
HypuroFit.com

Further Reading

While not directly quoted, the below list contains texts that have been formative in our thought and may be fruitful resources for those looking to explore the topics we covered more deeply.

Gaudium et Spes:
On the Church in the Modern World
Vatican Council II

Man and Woman He Created Them
Pope St. John Paul II

Love and Responsibility
Pope St. John Paul II

Transformed by Grace
Dom Wulstan Mork, O.S.B.

Ascent of Mount Carmel
St. John of the Cross

The Interior Castle
St. Theresa of Avila

The Fulfillment of All Desire
Ralph Martin

About Hypuro Fit

Hypuro Fit was born out of a friendship and a desire
to see the modern church be renewed through
a "baptism" of of the practice of exercise.

Caring for our spiritual health can never neglect
our physical health and too often we've seen bodily
care be completely ignored or indulged to excess.

Hypuro Fit exists to connect qualified and deeply
Catholic coaches with those looking to deepen
their experiene of prayer and exercise. This isn't
a program only for elite athletes, it's a message
for every person of every age and fitness level.

For more information visit us online
at *HypuroFit.com* or follow us on
Instagram or Facebook.

What does "Hypuro" even mean?

Great question!

Hypuro is just two Greek words that we
mashed together to capture the intensity
of the exercise experience and also reflect
its transformative components.

Hypomone is the Greek for steadfastness or
endurance and **pyr** is the word for fire. In effect, the
combined meaning is "I endure the fire". It's a phrase
that functions as a description - acknowledging the
unavoidable reality that life is struggle - and also
as a battle cry - a declaration of our acceptance.
That we stake our flag in that ground and overcome
it rather than let ourselves be overcome.

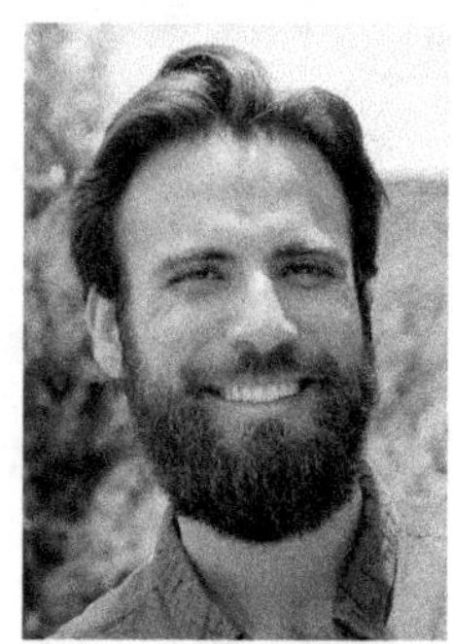

CHASE CROUSE

I began to see the connection of fitness and faith when I first had my reversion in 2012.

Fitness, and the grace of God, helped me to overcome my addictions because if I could mentally force my body to push itself and do something it didn't want to do, then I could stop myself from doing something that my body wanted to do in times of temptation. I later became a missionary with NET Ministries and have been in some form of apostolate ever since.

After pursuing my Undergraduate and Masters Degree in Theology my wife and I got married. While fitness was still important for me it wasn't until we got pregnant with our first child that I decided to pick up Personal Training to help supplement some income while my wife wasn't working. I ended up loving it!

I am a N.A.S.M. Certified Personal Trainer, an ACE Certified Functional Fitness Specialist, and Coach at OrangeTheory Fitness. My role at HypuroFit is to ensure that all of our programs are physically excellent, safe, and achievable, and that our spirituality is Orthodox and inspirational for all members.

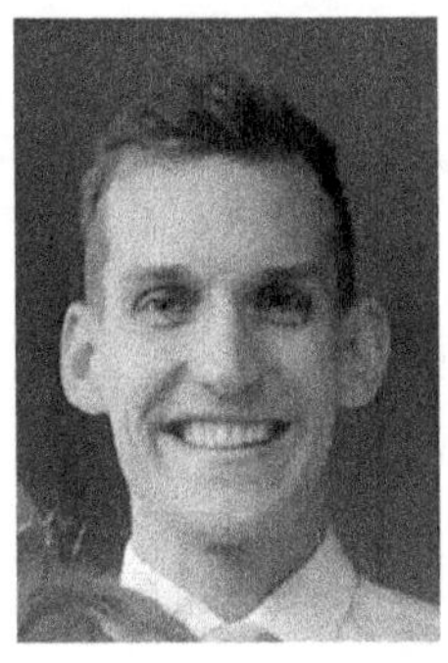

BEN WEST

I received my undergraduate B.S. in Media
Communications from John Paul the Great Catholic
University in Escondido, CA where I met Chase
and received much of my theological formation
under the instruction of Dr. Michael Barber,
Dr. John Kincaid, and Fr. Andrew Younan.

My interest in fitness blossomed alongisde my faith
in college. Nowadays my preferred form of torture
is obstacle races of which I am a finisher of the
Marine Bootcamp Challenge and Spartan Sprint.

I'm a motion designer by trade with a wide
range of creative skills and interests. As the
Operations Director of Hypuro Fit I oversee
our brand, messaging, online presence, and
most of our organizational components.

www.ingramcontent.com/pod-product-compliance
Lightning Source LLC
Chambersburg PA
CBHW052103150726
48002CB00006B/2206